Evaluation of Employee Exposure to Lead and Other Chemicals at a Police Department

Kenneth W. Fent, PhD, CIH
John Gibbins, DVM, MPH
Todd Niemeier, MS, CIH

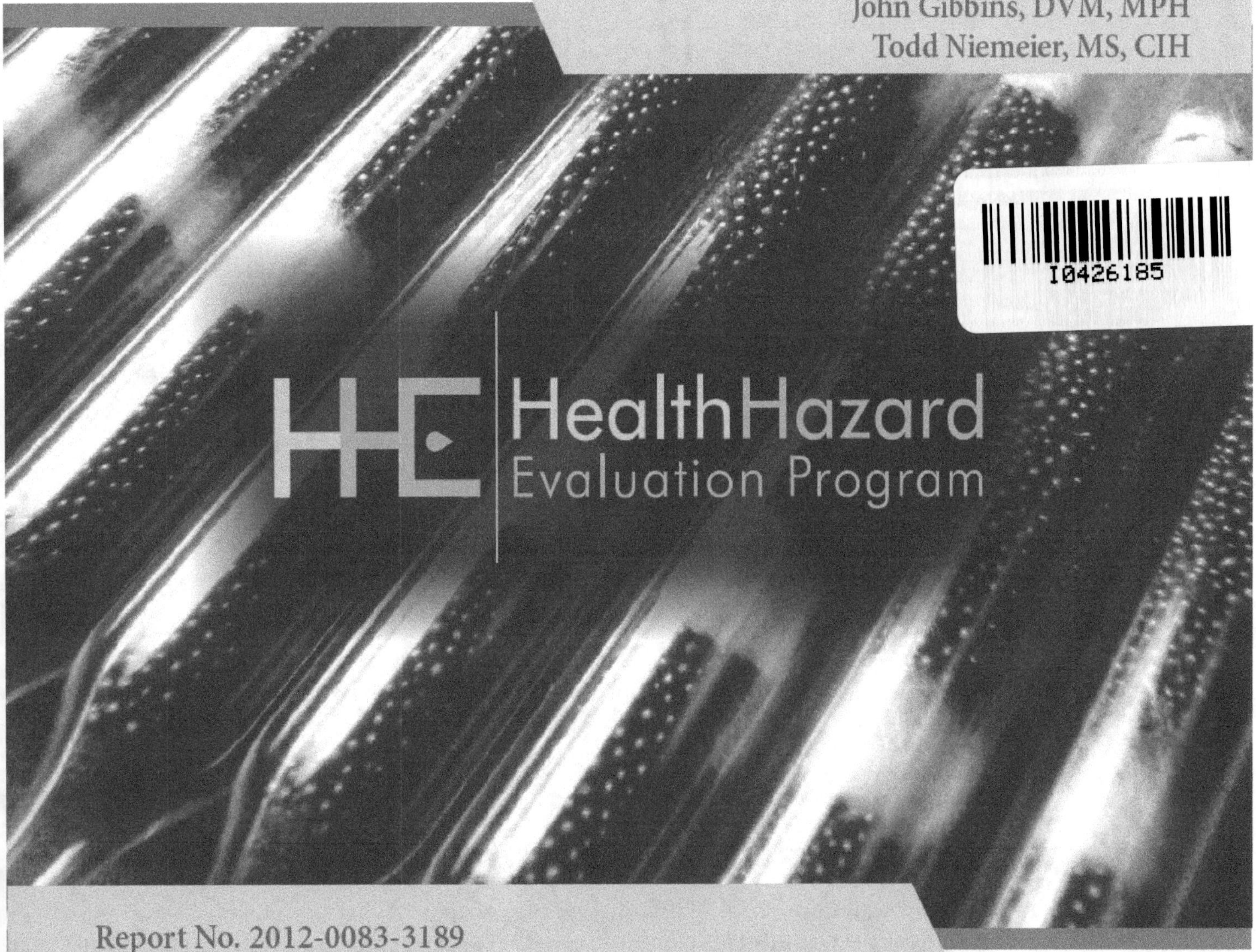

HealthHazard Evaluation Program

Report No. 2012-0083-3189
July 2013

U.S. Department of Health and Human Services
Centers for Disease Control and Prevention
National Institute for Occupational Safety and Health

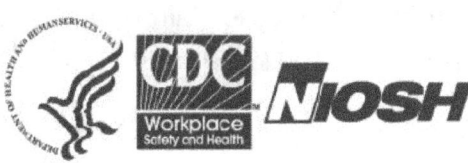

Contents

The cover photo is a close-up image of sorbent tubes, which are used by the HHE Program to measure airborne exposures. This photo is an artistic representation that may not be related to this Health Hazard Evaluation.

Highlights of this Evaluation

The Health Hazard Evaluation Program received a request from a police department in Ohio. Employees were concerned about exposure to lead from the firing range, mold in second floor offices, and ventilation in the illicit drug storage room.

What We Did

- We visited the facility in March and June 2012.

- We talked with employees about health concerns they related to work.

- We inspected the second floor ceiling for water intrusion and mold.

- We evaluated the firing range's ventilation and filtration system.

- We tested surfaces in the firing range and parking garage for lead.

- We tested surfaces in the property room for illicit drugs.

- We measured employee exposures to ethyl cyanoacrylate during cyanoacrylate fuming and carbon black during fingerprint dusting.

> We identified problems in the firing range ventilation system. We found lead contamination in the parking garage and illicit drug contamination in the property room. We recommend not using the firing range until its ventilation system has been redesigned and cleaning surfaces in the garage and property room.

What We Found

- Most employees we talked with had health symptoms they felt were related to the workplace.

- One employee had a higher than normal level of lead in his/her blood.

- We saw no signs of current water intrusion or mold.

- Air from the hallway and above the ceiling flowed into the second floor offices.

- The firing range did not meet all of the ventilation design elements recommended by the National Institute for Occupational Safety and Health.

- We found lead on surfaces inside the parking garage. The firing range was the main source of this lead.

- We found illicit drugs on some surfaces in the property room. Work surfaces had lower levels than undisturbed surfaces such as elevated shelving.

- We did not find ethyl cyanoacrylate vapor or carbon black particles in the air.

What the Employer Can Do

- Redesign the firing range or use another firing range that meets National Institute for Occupational Safety and Health recommendations. Do not use the firing range until it has been redesigned.

- Provide officers with non-lead bullets and lead-free primer.

- Sample the air for lead when officers use bullets or primer containing lead. Use the results to determine which elements of the Occupational Safety and Health Administration lead standard to follow.

- Clean surfaces where lead or illicit drugs were found.

- Hire a contractor to balance the second floor ventilation system.

- Set schedules for changing air filters in the local exhaust ventilation systems and vacuum cleaners.

- Start a health and safety committee that includes employee, employer, and union representatives. Hold regular meetings.

- Encourage employees to report health symptoms they think may be related to work.

What Employees Can Do

- Wear nitrile gloves when cleaning guns, handling spent cartridge cases, or working in the parking garage or firing range.

- Wear nitrile gloves when handling illicit drug evidence and doing criminology procedures.

- Clean hands with soap and water or with lead-decontamination wipes after firing guns or doing other work that could expose your hands to lead, even if you wear gloves.

- Become active in the health and safety committee.

- Report work-related health concerns to your supervisor.

Mention of any company or product does not constitute endorsement by NIOSH. In addition, citations to websites external to NIOSH do not constitute NIOSH endorsement of the sponsoring organizations or their programs or products. Furthermore, NIOSH is not responsible for the content of these websites. All web addresses referenced in this document were accessible as of the publication date of this report.

Abbreviations

$\mu g/100\ cm^2$	Micrograms per 100 square centimeters
$\mu g/ft^2$	Micrograms per square foot
$\mu g/dL$	Micrograms per deciliter
BLL	Blood lead level
cm	Centimeters
cm^2	Square centimeters
HEPA	High-efficiency particulate air
HUD	Department of Housing and Urban Development
HVAC	Heating, ventilating, and air-conditioning
MERV	Minimum efficiency reporting value
mm	Millimeters
ND	Not detected
$ng/100\ cm^2$	Nanograms per 100 square centimeters
NIOSH	National Institute for Occupational Safety and Health
OEL	Occupational exposure limit
OSHA	Occupational Safety and Health Administration
THC	Tetrahydrocannabinol

Introduction

The Health Hazard Evaluation Program received a request from employees at a police department in Ohio. The request concerned lead exposures in and around the firing range, a history of water intrusion and mold growth on the ceiling tiles in the juvenile office, and lack of ventilation in the property room where illicit drugs were stored. We made two site visits to the police department to evaluate exposures, work conditions, and employee health concerns.

The police department was in a two-story building. Our evaluation focused mainly on the second floor and basement. The second floor contained offices (including the juvenile office) and a crime lab. The basement contained a parking garage, property room, and firing range.

The juvenile office had a drop ceiling with tiles that were reported to have mold growth at one time. The juvenile office was staffed by three to four officers, mainly during the first shift. The crime lab was in a section of the old jail. Two box fans had been strapped to the windows in the crime lab to provide exhaust ventilation by directing air outdoors. The crime lab had a Sirchie model FR600 cyanoacrylate fuming chamber with a recirculating high-efficiency particulate air (HEPA) filter and a DeFumigator™ model FR300 carbon-bed filtration system, a Mystaire Misonix tabletop exhaust hood with recirculating carbon-bed filtration, and a Microzone Corporation model EPH-2-4 fingerprint powder downdraft table with HEPA filtration. The crime lab was used by one or two officers, and generally for no more than a few hours per week.

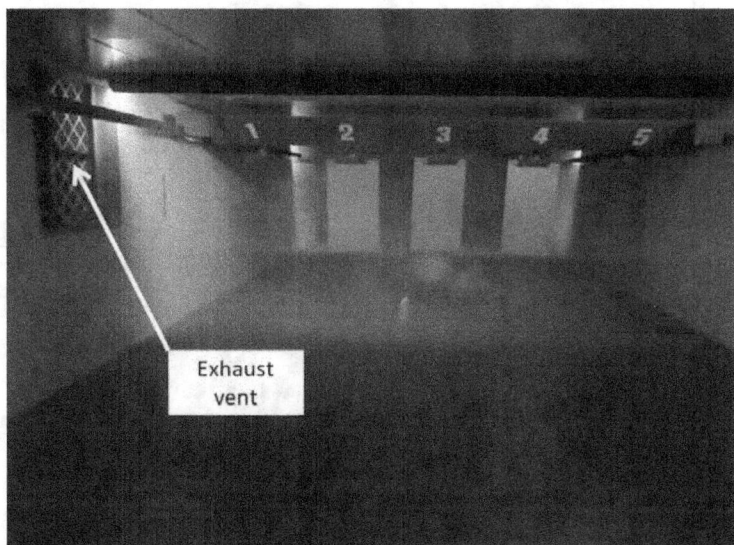

Figure 1. Inside of firing range.

The firing range was next to the parking garage. It had five lanes, but only the three center lanes (lanes 2–4) were used for weapons qualifications (Figure 1). The range dimensions were 86 feet deep × 19 feet wide × 7.5 feet tall. Equipment and tables were placed along the walls uprange and downrange (in the areas of lanes 1 and 5). The firing line was 16 feet from the rear wall. Five ceiling-mounted supply air diffusers were positioned 7 feet behind the firing line. Air was exhausted from the range via a sidewall exhaust ventilation system 32 feet downrange from the firing line (38 feet uprange of the bullet trap). The exhaust ventilation filtration system (Figure 2) contained a minimum efficiency reporting value (MERV)-8 pre-filter and MERV-14 primary filter.

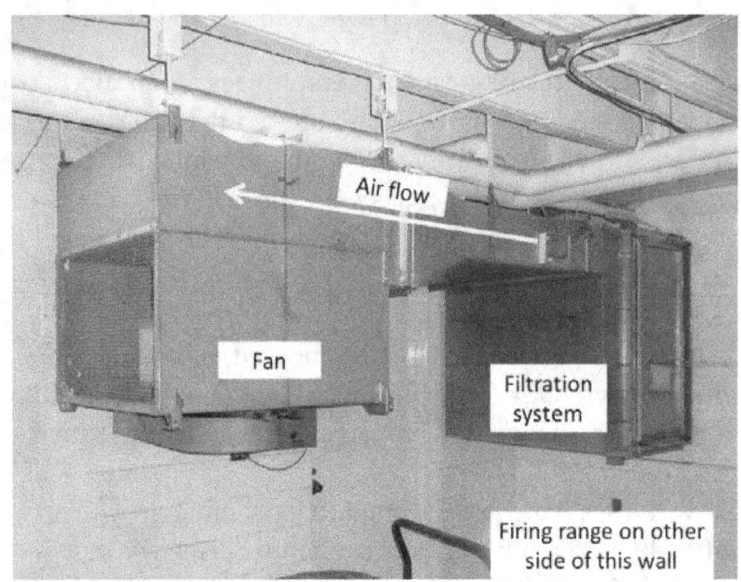

Figure 2. Exhaust ventilation system for the firing range that discharges air into the parking garage.

The exhaust air discharged directly into the garage. The prefilter was changed quarterly, and the primary filter was changed biannually by a heating, ventilating, and air-conditioning (HVAC) contractor.

Approximately 100 officers used the firing range. Officers reported that targets were placed downrange of the exhaust fan and that officers stood at the firing line directly adjacent to the exhaust fan to fire their weapons. Officers qualified one time per year by firing 60 rounds with a handgun and shotgun. Duty ammunition that contained lead was used for qualification. At all other times, clean-fire ammunition containing lead-free primer and a total metal jacket was used. After several qualifications, the department's bomb team used a Nilfisk model CFM S2 HEPA vacuum to clean the floors and bullet trap in the range while wearing a DuPont™ Tyvek® suit and a respirator. The employer did not know the type of respirator worn. A range officer emptied the dust collected by the vacuum as needed. Officers reported that personal protective equipment was not worn when emptying the vacuum.

The property room was also adjacent to the parking garage. The property room did not contain an exhaust ventilation system, but did have a recirculating ceiling-mounted steam heater and a wall-mounted air-conditioning unit. One or two officers could spend 2 hours or more per day inside the property room documenting, storing, retrieving, or inventorying criminal evidence. The automotive maintenance employee's office was also adjacent to the garage. This employee maintained the patrol vehicles parked in the garage.

Methods

During our March 2012 visit we met with employer and employee representatives to discuss the health hazard evaluation request. The police department provided us with a copy of a consultant's lead assessment in the firing range and parking garage and the HVAC contractor's report summarizing the preventive maintenance on the HVAC system. We held confidential interviews with 12 of 15 employees who worked in the firing range, basement property room and maintenance areas, and second floor juvenile and detective offices and administrative areas. We asked about their work history, health concerns, medical history, and the department's occupational health surveillance program. We reviewed medical records from two of five employees who reported seeking medical care for their symptoms.

During the March 2012 visit we inspected the plenum (the space above the suspended ceiling) in the juvenile office and other second floor offices for evidence of water intrusion or mold growth. Because the ceiling tiles in the juvenile office were sealed, we removed a ceiling tile in the adjacent waiting area and used a Fluke® Ti55 FlexCam thermal imaging camera to identify cooler areas in the ceiling as an indicator of water damage or water intrusion. We inspected the firing range and its exhaust ventilation system. We used Gastec Corporation ventilation smoke tubes to visualize the movement of gun smoke within the firing range. We also used a TSI condensation particle counter in the parking garage approximately 20 feet downstream from the exhaust ventilation discharge grilles to measure airborne submicron particulate levels while the firing range was in use. For comparison, we measured the particulate in the exhaust air when the firing range was not in use. We used SKC Inc. Full Disclosure® colorimetric wipes to test surfaces in the firing range, garage, and automotive maintenance office for lead contamination. These wipes produce a color change if lead is present. We measured relative humidity and airflow direction (relative to adjacent areas) in the property room and second floor office area. Relative humidity was measured with a TSI Q-trak™ Plus, and airflow direction was determined with a Gastec Corporation ventilation smoke tube. Finally, an officer showed us the crime lab in the old jail where criminology equipment and techniques were used.

On the basis of our March 2012 findings we returned to the police department in June 2012 to evaluate in more detail the exhaust ventilation and filtration system in the firing range, lead contamination in the basement, and potential illicit drug contamination in the property room. We also sampled the air for ethyl cyanoacrylate during cyanoacrylate fuming inside the crime lab and carbon black particulate (a component of Sirchie HI-FI silk black fingerprint powder) during fingerprint dusting of a vehicle inside the parking garage. The officer who did the cyanoacrylate fuming wore nitrile gloves when handling the cyanoacrylate strips. The officer who did the fingerprint dusting wore nitrile gloves and a National Institute for Occupational Safety and Health (NIOSH)-approved N95 filtering facepiece respirator (3M model 1860). Table 1 provides a summary of the surface and air sampling methods we used during our June 2012 visit. Templates (10 centimeters × 10 centimeters) were used for sampling flat surfaces. For irregularly shaped surfaces, we estimated approximately 100 square centimeters (cm^2) and wiped the surface in a manner similar to that used for flat surfaces.

Table 1. Summary of the air and surface sampling methods used in June 2012

Analyte(s)	Sampling media	Flow rate or surface area	Method	No. of samples
Surface sampling				
Lead	SKC Full Disclosure® wipes	100 cm^2	Colorimetric change and NIOSH 7303*	18
Illicit drugs (heroin, THC, methamphetamine, and cocaine)	Cotton swab prewetted with buffer solution	100 cm^2	Microbead immunosorbent assay [Smith et al. 2010]	12
Air sampling				
Ethyl cyanoacrylate	XAD-7 sorbent tube	0.2 Lpm	OSHA 55†	5‡
Carbon black	25-mm IOM sampler with preweighed PVC filter	2 Lpm	NIOSH 0600*	1§
	BGI 4L respirable dust cyclone¶, 37-mm cassette with preweighed PVC filter	2.2 Lpm	NIOSH 0500*	1§

IOM = Institute of Medicine

Lpm = liters per minute

mm = millimeters

PVC = polyvinylchloride

THC = tetrahydrocannabinol

*NIOSH Manual of Analytical Methods [NIOSH 2013]

†Occupational Safety and Health Administration (OSHA) Sampling and Analytical Methods [OSHA 1985]

‡Collected three area air samples and two personal air samples worn by one officer during cyanoacrylate fuming of evidence.

§Personal air samplers worn by one officer on the same shoulder during fingerprint dusting of a vehicle.

¶BGI Incorporated (Waltham, Massachusetts)

To evaluate the ventilation system in the firing range we used an aerosol generating machine (Rosco Laboratories Inc. model 1500) to generate "theatrical smoke" (actually a submicron liquid aerosol). The smoke was used to visualize airflow patterns in each of the firing lanes. Smoke was generated at four points along the length of the range: the firing line, 17 feet downrange, 32 feet downrange, and at the bullet trap. We also used a TSI VelociCalc® Plus air velocity meter to measure airflow at the firing line and at three points downrange from the firing line (17 feet, 32 feet, and at the bullet trap). Triplicate measurements were collected in each lane along the firing line at two different heights (approximately 3 feet and 5 feet). These measurements were averaged and the average was reported for each location.

To test the effectiveness of the filtration system in the firing range we used a TSI condensation particle counter in the parking garage approximately 20 feet downstream from the exhaust grilles. We measured airborne submicron particle levels in the exhaust while theatrical smoke was generated in the firing range. For comparison, we measured the particulate in the exhaust air when the firing range was clear of theatrical smoke.

Results and Discussion

Employee Interviews and Symptoms

The average length of employment at the department was 20 years (range: 8 to 36 years). Eight of 12 (67%) employees reported symptoms they felt were related to work. Approximately one third of interviewed employees reported shortness of breath, sneezing, sinus congestion, and itchy eyes. Most employees stated their symptoms improved on days off or when not working on the second floor. Some employees reported seasonal allergies that were also associated with nonwork exposures. Multiple factors could contribute to these nonspecific symptoms. These factors include prior mold exposure, poor indoor environmental quality, and discomfort due to fluctuations in temperature and humidity. Some employees may have been more sensitive to these factors than others, and thus more likely to report symptoms. Nonwork exposures and seasonal allergies can also contribute to symptoms.

Five employees previously sought medical care for health effects they thought could be work-related. Four of these employees were seen for symptoms attributed to recurring allergies, sinus infections, and chronic back pain. An employee who worked in the basement sought medical care for fatigue, headache, and leg weakness/pain. This employee's blood was tested for lead as part of a medical evaluation. The employee's blood lead level (BLL) was 38 micrograms per deciliter (μg/dL). After sharing the test results with the employer, this employee was moved to the second floor. The employee's BLL gradually decreased to 5.7 μg/dL over the next 8 months.

An employee's BLL should be maintained below 40 μg/dL according to OSHA [29 CFR 1910.1025] and below 30 μg/dL according to the American Conference of Governmental Industrial Hygienists [ACGIH 2013]. These levels are intended to prevent overt symptoms of lead poisoning; the OSHA recommendations were set almost 30 years ago. Controlling lead at these levels has not been found to be sufficient to protect employees from more subtle adverse health effects including high blood pressure, kidney problems, reproductive concerns such as infertility, and cognitive effects [Schwartz and Hu 2007; Schwartz and Stewart 2007; Brown-Williams et al. 2009]. Acute lead poisoning is uncommon today due to current occupational exposure limits (OELs). Acute lead poisoning, with BLLs usually over 70 μg/dL, can result in clinical symptoms such as abdominal pain, hemolytic anemia, and neuropathy, and in very rare cases has progressed to encephalopathy and coma [Moline and Landrigan 2005]. Chronic lead poisoning may not cause any symptoms, or may present with a variety of symptoms including headache, joint and muscle aches, weakness, fatigue, irritability, depression, constipation, anorexia, and abdominal discomfort [Moline and Landrigan 2005]. The non-specific symptoms of headache, fatigue, and leg pain in this employee have been reported with chronic lead exposure and BLLs of 40–50 μg/dL or lower in individuals with other medical conditions. We do not know how this employee's BLL had been elevated or if it was ever higher than 38 μg/dL. Overexposure to lead may also result in kidney damage, anemia, high blood pressure, infertility and reduced sex drive in both sexes, and impotence in men.

A panel of experts published guidelines to prevent both acute and chronic effects of lead poisoning in adults [Kosnett et al. 2007]. It recommended removing an employee from exposure if a single BLL exceeds 30 µg/dL, or if two measurements taken over 4 weeks exceed 20 µg/dL. Removal should be considered if control measures over an extended period do not decrease BLLs to < 10 µg/dL. The panel also recommended quarterly BLL testing if the BLL is between 10 and 19 µg/dL, and semiannual testing if the BLL is < 10 µg/dL. Pregnant women should avoid BLLs > 5 µg/dL. These guidelines are endorsed by the California Department of Public Health and the Council of State and Territorial Epidemiologists [California Department of Public Health 2009; CSTE 2009]. The NIOSH adult blood lead reference value is 10 µg/dL. The NIOSH Adult Blood Lead Epidemiology and Surveillance program tracks elevated BLLs (i.e., BLLs at or above the reference values) among adults in the United States. The geometric mean BLL among adults age 20 and older in the United States is 1.23 µg/dL [CDC 2013]. The CDC recommends public health actions when the BLL in children is 5 µg/dL or higher. This "reference level" identifies children ages 1–5 years in the United States whose BLLs are higher than 97.5% of children based on the National Health and Nutrition Examination Survey, and is designed to allow early action be taken to reduce further exposure to lead [CDC 2012].

Occupational exposure to inorganic lead occurs via inhalation of lead-containing dust and fume and ingestion of lead particles from contact with lead-contaminated surfaces. In cases where careful attention to hygiene (for example, hand washing) is not practiced, smoking cigarettes or eating may represent another route of exposure among employees who are exposed to lead and then transfer it to their mouth through hand contamination.

Occupational exposures can also create non-occupational exposures among household members, including children, from take-home contamination with lead. Take-home contamination occurs when lead dust is transferred from an employee's skin, clothing, shoes, and other personal items to their vehicle.

In addition to their health symptoms, employees told us they did not receive annual audiograms or blood lead tests; this was confirmed by the employer. OSHA requires annual audiometric testing if an employee's full-shift time-weighted average exposure level is ≥ 85 A-weighted decibels [29 CFR 1910.95]. Although we did not evaluate noise exposures, evaluations at other indoor firing ranges have found peak sound pressure levels > 155 decibels [Kardous et al. 2003; NIOSH 2003; Murphy and Tubbs 2007]; exposures to these extreme sound levels for just a few seconds or less will result in full-shift time-weighted average exposures ≥ 85 A-weighted decibels. Studies have shown that exposure to lead can enhance noise-induced hearing loss [Hwang et al. 2009]. The U.S. Army recommends annual audiometric testing if employees are exposed to lead at levels ≥ 50% of the most protective OEL [U.S. Army 2009].

Many employees expressed concern about the cleaning, maintenance, and operation of the HVAC system, as well as previous roof leaks and mold growth on the second floor that they felt contributed to their symptoms. Several employees stated that desk surfaces, supply air vents in offices, and the maintenance room had been cleaned prior to our first visit. Employees also mentioned that areas of the range had recently been painted and the employer had recently purchased a HEPA vacuum for cleaning the range. The employer stated that part-time cleaning services were provided by the city under contract, and these services were typically only available from 9:00 a.m. to 5:00 p.m. According to the employer, general maintenance and repair of the building was the responsibility of the city.

Second Floor Offices: Mold Inspection

We found no evidence of current water intrusion or visible mold contamination on the ceiling tiles or the plenum area of the second floor offices. Because we had only a limited view of the plenum area above the juvenile office, we cannot be certain that no mold was present. Past water intrusion, however, was evident from water-stained ceiling tiles. According to an HVAC contractor's report, no microbial contamination or mechanical problems were found in the HVAC system inspection. Using ventilation smoke tubes, we found that the second floor office area was under negative pressure relative to the hallway and plenum (meaning that air was flowing from the hallway and plenum and into the office area). The large volume of air coming from the plenum and hallway suggested that the HVAC system needed balancing. The relative humidity was 50% in the second floor offices during our March 2012 visit. However, we only sampled during 1 day in the early spring. Humidity levels are likely to vary over time. The American Industrial Hygiene Association recommends maintaining relative humidity below 60% to minimize microbial growth [AIHA 2010].

Firing Range: Ventilation Assessment and Noise Considerations

A summary of the ventilation flow rate measurements is provided in Table 2. The firing range did not meet the NIOSH recommendations for supply air ventilation design [NIOSH 2009]. Most notably, some airflow rates along the firing line exceeded the NIOSH maximum recommended airflow of 75 feet per minute. Excessive air velocities can cause eddies (air currents that run contrary to the main current). A few of our ventilation measurements 17 feet downrange and all of our ventilation measurements at the bullet trap were below the NIOSH minimum recommended airflow of 30 feet per minute that is intended to minimize the fallout of gun emissions downrange. Overall, the airflow was not evenly distributed across the firing range. This can result in a reversal of airflow. We visualized this reverse airflow in the firing range using theatrical smoke and found the following:

- Smoke generated at the firing line traveled downrange, reversed direction, and then traveled back towards the firing line.

- Smoke generated 17 feet downrange of the firing line traveled downrange toward the exhaust fan.

- Smoke generated 32 feet downrange traveled downrange, reversed direction back toward the smoke generation point, and then exhausted from the range.

- Smoke generated at the bullet trap traveled uprange toward the exhaust fan and was exhausted from the range.

The firing range did not meet many of the NIOSH recommendations for exhaust ventilation

Table 2. Firing range ventilation flow rates (feet per minute) measured during the second visit

Firing lane	Firing line		Downrange (17 feet)		Downrange (32 feet)		Bullet trap	
	3 feet height	5 feet height	3 feet height	5 feet height	3 feet height	5 feet height	3 feet height	5 feet height
2	51	95	46	21	32	35	4	13
3	162	70	30	31	35	48	4	7
4	281	205	68	15	39	42	3	3
Mean	165	123	48	22	35	42	4	8
Overall mean	144		35		39		6	

design [NIOSH 2009]. Most notably, the air should be exhausted at or behind the bullet trap, not from the sidewall halfway down the range. The air should also be exhausted outdoors after being filtered with a HEPA or MERV-18/19 primary filter. These filters capture a minimum of 99.97% of 0.3-micron diameter particles, which is the most difficult particle size to capture [EPA 2009]. The air at this firing range was exhausted indoors (in the garage) and was filtered with a MERV-14 primary filter that only captures 75%–85% of 0.3-micron diameter particles [EPA 2009]. This explains why we were able to detect submicron particles in the firing range exhaust when the range was in use or filled with theatrical smoke. Figure 3 shows elevated submicron particle concentrations (compared to background levels) in the exhaust air during and shortly after an officer fired several shots from a 9-mm handgun in the firing range during our first visit. The ammunition used in this gun contained non-lead primer and a total metal jacket bullet. However, even when lead-free ammunition is used, other potentially harmful metal particulate can be produced (depending on the makeup of the bullet). Figure 4 shows elevated submicron particle concentrations (compared to background levels) in the exhaust air when we generated theatrical smoke in the firing range during our second visit.

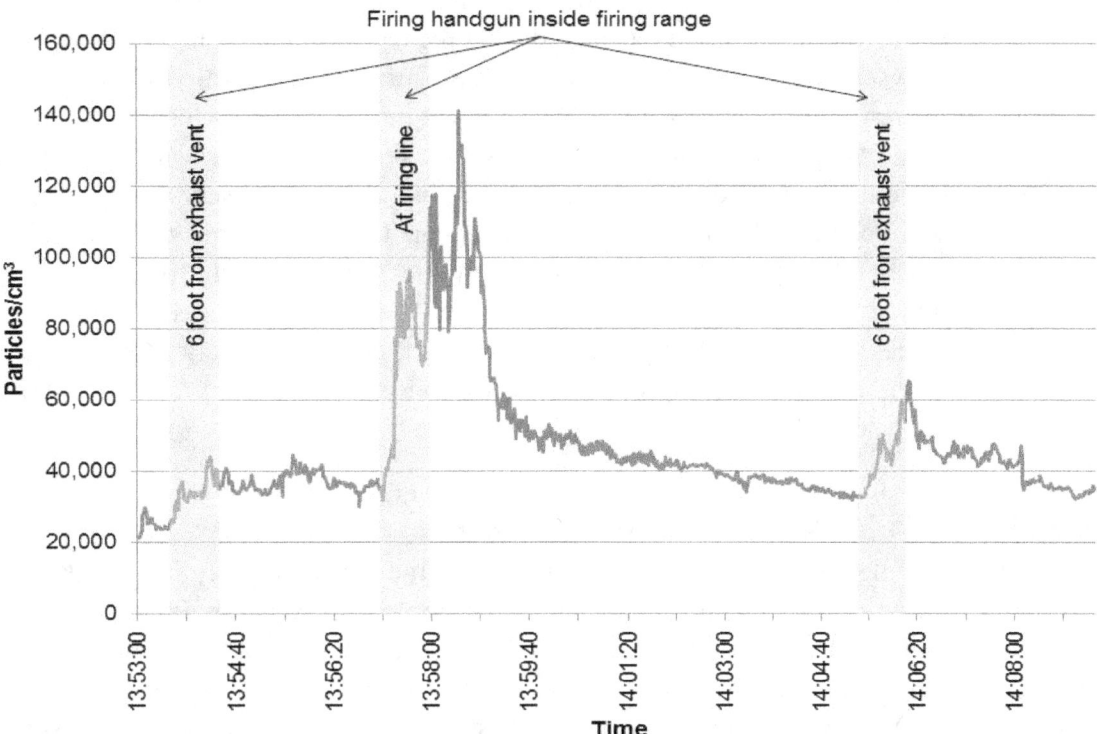

Figure 3. Submicron particle number concentrations measured in the exhaust air of the firing range while an officer fired his weapon inside the firing range during the first visit.

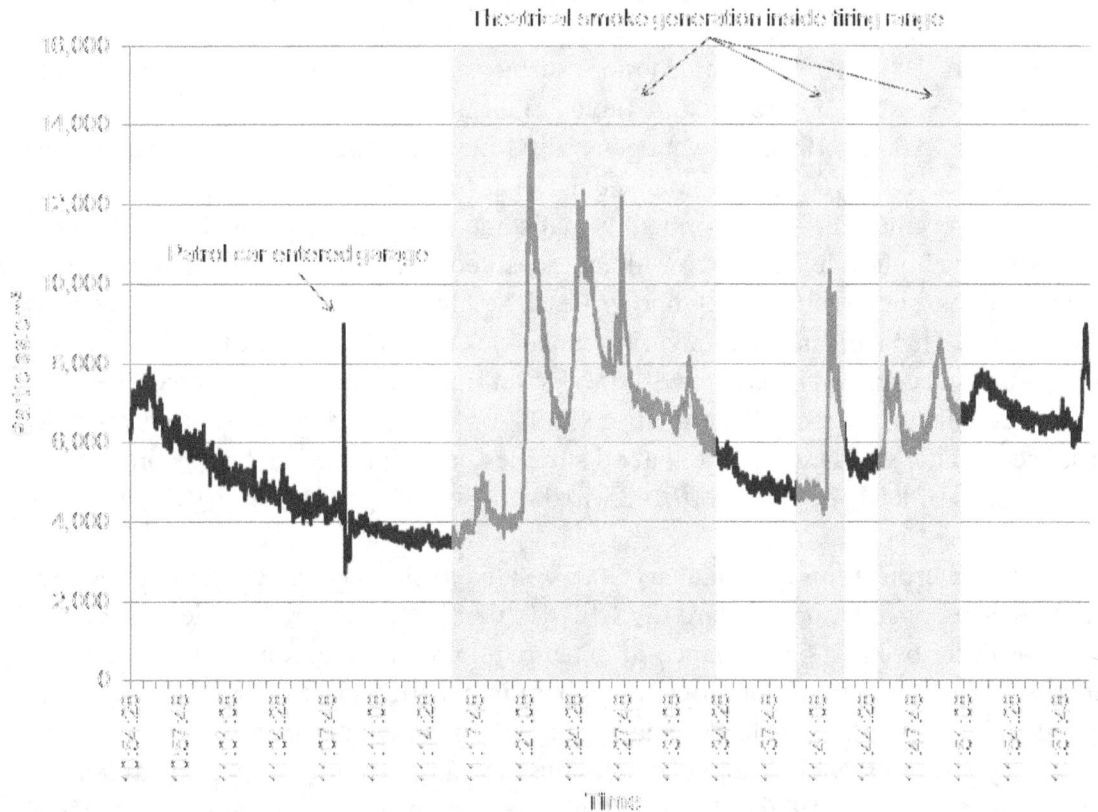

Figure 4. Submicron particle number concentrations measured in the exhaust air of the firing range while theatrical smoke was generated inside the firing range during the second visit.

Noise-induced hearing loss is one of the most common occupational diseases [NIOSH 2001]. Although we did not monitor noise exposures during the evaluation, employees were exposed to impulse noise when firing weapons. While their exposures were typically of short duration, prolonged exposures to impulse noise may lead to noise-induced hearing loss [Chan et al. 2001]. According to the police department, officers were required to wear earmuffs during shooting. However, none of the officers were included in a hearing conservation program. NIOSH has made recommendations for preventing occupational exposures to noise at indoor firing ranges [NIOSH 2009]. NIOSH recommends engineering, administrative, and personal protective equipment measures to limit noise exposure. These recommendations include requiring employees who use the firing range to wear dual hearing protection (ear plugs and earmuffs) and enrolling these employees in a hearing conservation program that adheres to the OSHA noise standard [29 CFR 1910.95].

Parking Garage: Lead Contamination

In the past, lead bullets and primers had been used for practice and qualifying rounds. The new policy required clean-fire ammunition (non-lead primer and total metal jacket bullet) for all practice rounds. Duty ammunition was still required for qualifying rounds. Some of the lead particles produced by firearms during past practices (or during more recent qualifying rounds) likely passed through the exhaust filtration system and were deposited into the parking garage. During our first visit we found qualitative evidence (i.e., color change indications) of lead contamination on the exhaust grilles inside the garage and on the door handle and computer mouse inside the automotive maintenance office. The approximate level that can be detected by color change is 18 micrograms per 100 square centimeters ($\mu g/100$ cm^2). We sampled more surfaces during our second visit; the qualitative and quantitative results are provided in Table 3. Our measurements (ranging from 1.8 $\mu g/100$ cm^2 to 3,100 $\mu g/100$ cm^2) were generally lower than the consultant's measurements made approximately 1 year prior to our second visit (ranging from 1,200 $\mu g/100$ cm^2 to 210,000 $\mu g/100$ cm^2). Officers informed us that some surfaces had been cleaned before our evaluation. The highest levels the consultant measured were in the firing range and in the garage at or near the exhaust ventilation grilles. The highest levels we measured were also in these areas. This indicates that the firing range was the main source of lead contamination in the garage. Occupational health and safety government agencies or national organizations have not established surface contamination limits for lead. However, OSHA specifies in its substance-specific standard for lead that all surfaces be maintained as free as practicable of accumulations of lead [29 CFR 1910.1025(h)(1)].

In a letter of interpretation from January 2003 related to surface lead contamination in the OSHA lead-in-construction standard [29 CFR 1926.62], "free as practicable of accumulations of lead" is described as a performance-oriented requirement. According to OSHA, "The requirement is met when the employer is vigilant in his efforts to ensure that surfaces are kept free of accumulations of lead-containing dust. The intent of this provision is to ensure that employers regularly clean and conduct housekeeping activities to prevent avoidable lead exposure" [29 CFR 1926.62]. To evaluate the effectiveness of cleaning in change areas, storage facilities, and lunchrooms/eating areas, OSHA recommends using the Department of Housing and Urban Development (HUD) acceptable decontamination level for lead of 200 micrograms per square foot ($\mu g/ft^2$) for floors [OSHA 2003].

Since the time that OSHA issued this letter of interpretation, HUD lowered the acceptable decontamination level for lead to 40 $\mu g/ft^2$ for carpeted and noncarpeted horizontal surfaces [HUD 2012]. To our knowledge, OSHA has not determined whether the lower HUD decontamination level should be considered a concentration of lead in workplaces that is "free as practicable of accumulations of lead." Because we measured lead contamination on an area of 100 cm^2, our results are not directly comparable to the HUD decontamination levels (measured on an area of 1 square foot or about 930 cm^2). Assuming that the lead was equally distributed on the surfaces we sampled, then some of our surface measurements may exceed the HUD decontamination level of 200 $\mu g/ft^2$ (22 $\mu g/100$ cm^2), including surfaces inside the parking garage. Ultimately, the police department will need to determine what it believes represents "free as practicable of accumulations of lead."

Table 3. Qualitative and quantitative sampling results for surface contamination of lead during the second visit

General location	Specific location	Qualitative result	Quantitative result ($\mu g/100$ cm^2)†
Evidence room	Door vent inside room	+	88
	Computer desk	+	(4.5)
	Table next to computer	+	(1.8)
	Metal cart	+	34
Firing range	Floor	+	3,100
	Table	+	490
Parking garage	Desk next to elevator	−	(1.9)
	Upper corner of the firing range exhaust vent	+	2,200
	Floor by range exit	+	2,600
	Steering wheel of patrol car (window open)	−	(4.9)
	Floor outside the elevator	+	32
	Floor by bicycles	+	170
	Bicycle handles	+	28
	Door knob to mechanic room	+	23
Mechanic room	Middle table	+	14
	Desk	+	16
Second floor	Outside elevator	+	44
	Computer mouse in the range officer's office	−	(5.4)
Detection limit			0.3
Quantitation limit			8.0

*Color change = "+" or positive for lead. No color change = "−" or negative for lead.

†Values between the detection limit and quantitation limit are shown in parentheses to point out that there is more uncertainty associated with these values than with levels above the quantitation limit.

Local government agencies like police departments are not regulated by OSHA. Nevertheless, OSHA regulations or more protective guidelines should be followed to protect the health and safety of employees. The OSHA lead standard [29 CFR 1910.1025] requires each employer who operates a firing range to determine if any employees may be exposed to lead at or above the action level (30 micrograms per cubic meter of air as an 8-hour time-weighted average). The employer is also required to institute a medical surveillance program, including biological monitoring, for employees who are exposed to lead at or above the action level for > 30 days per year. We did not do air sampling for lead because the firing range was used infrequently during our visit. Because we observed reverse air flow in the range and because air from the firing range was exhausted into the parking garage, the range officer and automotive maintenance employee (who works in the garage) may have the greatest potential for exposure to lead at or above the action level. After the second site visit in June 2012, we recommended that the police department stop using the firing range because (1) it did not meet NIOSH design recommendations [NIOSH 2009] and (2) it was contaminating the garage with lead and possibly exposing employees. As of June 2013, the police department was still using the firing range.

Property Room: Illicit Drug and Mold Contamination

Table 4 presents the levels of illicit drugs measured on surfaces in the property room. Other than for cocaine, the levels were mostly not detected (ND) or below the quantitation limit. The cocaine levels measured on work surfaces, such as the computer desk or front table, were lower than the levels measured on undisturbed areas such as the corner of table 2 or the shelf above the computer desk. Occupational health and safety government agencies or national organizations have not established surface contamination limits for illicit drugs. However, several states have established feasibility-based surface contamination limits when remediating clandestine laboratories for methamphetamine ranging from 100 nanograms per 100 square centimeters (ng/100 cm^2) to 500 ng/100 cm^2 [NAMSDL 2008]. The methamphetamine levels we measured were below the detection limit of 10 ng/100 cm^2. In the past, we sampled surfaces for illicit drugs during an evaluation of a drug vault at another police department and found on average higher levels of THC, methamphetamine, and cocaine (heroin was not sampled) than what we measured in this evaluation [NIOSH 2011]. Although acute and chronic health effects from the low levels of drugs found in the property room appear unlikely, we cannot definitively state that they did not contribute in part to reported symptoms. Additionally, potential exposure to illicit drugs stored as evidence will likely vary over time and may be higher during periods of increased work load .and evidence processing.

Table 4. Surface contamination levels of illicit drugs in the property room (ng/100 cm²)

Location	Heroin*	THC*	Cocaine*	Methamphetamine
Front table	(1.7)	ND	49	ND
Table 2 in the rear of the room	(1.5)	ND	150	ND
Corner of table 2	(1.4)	(2.7)	270	ND
Top of ladder	(1.1)	ND	170	ND
Cart, second shelf from top	(1.0)	ND	51	ND
Inside secure narcotics cabinet	ND	ND	71	ND
Floor in front of narcotics cabinet	ND	ND	140	ND
Computer mouse	(1.4)	ND	ND	ND
Computer desk	(1.4)	ND	(35)	ND
Shelf above computer desk	11	ND	290	ND
Ear piece of phone	(1.1)	ND	ND	ND
Floor under marijuana cage	ND	4.4	170	ND
Limit of detection per sample	0.9	2	20	10
Limit of quantitation per sample	1.9	3.2	38	21

*Values between the detection limit and quantitation limit are shown in parentheses to point out that there is more uncertainty associated with these values than with levels above the quantitation limit.

The property room was under slight positive pressure relative to the adjacent garage during the first visit. The American Society of Heating, Refrigerating, and Air-Conditioning Engineers does not provide specific exhaust ventilation flow rate recommendations for drug vaults or property rooms other than that they should be kept under negative pressure [ASHRAE 2007]. This recommendation is mainly intended to keep odors (e.g., marijuana odors) or volatile contaminants from migrating to adjacent occupied spaces. However, engine exhaust in the garage likely presented a greater health hazard than the marijuana odors, which are mostly terpenes [Lai et al. 2008; NIOSH 2011]. Few terpenes have occupational exposure limits. Therefore, it may be better to keep the property room under positive pressure. The relative humidity inside the property room during our March 2012 visit was 55%. The American Industrial Hygiene Association recommends maintaining relative humidity below 60% to minimize microbial growth [AIHA 2010]. We did not see any visual evidence of mold growing on the paper bags and cardboard boxes that held marijuana or other plant-based drugs.

Criminology Procedures: Potential Chemical Exposures

The minimum detectable concentrations for the compounds we sampled in air were calculated by dividing the detection limit for each compound by the average volume of air sampled. The minimum detectable concentrations represent the smallest air concentrations that could have been detected on the basis of volume of air sampled.

All the personal and area air concentrations of ethyl cyanoacrylate measured during cyanoacrylate fuming were ND (below the minimum detectable concentration of 0.024 parts per million). This procedure lasted and was sampled for about 40 minutes. One area air sample collected between the two exhaust fans was excluded because the sampling pump malfunctioned. The American Conference of Governmental Industrial Hygienists threshold limit value for ethyl cyanoacrylate is 0.2 parts per million (as an 8-hour time-weighted average) [ACGIH 2013] and is based upon the potential for eye, skin, and upper respiratory tract irritation; dermatitis; and possible respiratory sensitization or asthma [ACGIH 2001]. Although the threshold limit value does not have a skin notation, skin contact has been shown to cause adhesions that result in tissue damage [ACGIH 2001]. Our sampling results suggest that if cyanoacrylate fuming was performed for an entire 8-hour work shift, the air concentrations would not exceed the threshold limit value. This assumes, however, that the cyanoacrylate filtration system would perform optimally over the entire shift. If the carbon-bed filter were to become saturated, then higher airborne concentrations of ethyl cyanoacrylate concentrations would be expected.

The personal air concentrations of respirable and inhalable carbon black measured during the dusting of a car were ND (below the minimum detectable concentration of 2.0 milligrams per cubic meter). This procedure lasted and was sampled for about 25 minutes. The OSHA permissible exposure limit and NIOSH recommended exposure limit for carbon black are 3.5 milligrams per cubic meter as an (8 to 10-hour time-weighted average) [NIOSH 2010]. The threshold limit value for carbon black is 3 milligrams per cubic meter (as an 8-hour time-weighted average) [ACGIH 2013]. These OELs are primarily intended to minimize the irritation and inflammation of the respiratory system [NIOSH 2010; ACGIH 2011]. NIOSH set a lower recommended exposure limit for carbon black containing polycyclic aromatic hydrocarbons [NIOSH 2010]. However, fingerprint powder generally contains commercial-grade carbon black that should not contain polycyclic aromatic hydrocarbons. In a previous evaluation of another crime lab, the same type of powder used by this department (Sirchie HI-FI silk black) was found not to contain polycyclic aromatic hydrocarbons [NIOSH 2011].

Our sampling results suggest that if fingerprint dusting of a car were performed for an entire 8-hour work shift, the air concentrations would not exceed the applicable OELs. However, the officer who did the dusting was tall (> 6 feet in height). A shorter officer's breathing zone would be closer to the dusting area, and therefore higher personal air concentrations of carbon black would be expected. Fingerprint dusting of other objects or at a crime scene could result in different concentrations of carbon black than what we measured.

During a survey at another police department, we analyzed four commonly used powders, including Sirchie HI-FI silk black, and found that these powders were primarily composed of submicron particles [unpublished data]. Recent research suggests that inhalation of smaller carbon black particles may be more likely to cause pulmonary inflammation than large carbon black particles [Ward et al. 2010]. This is why we measured inhalable and respirable carbon black. Inhalable particles are large (up to 100-micron diameter or larger) and can be deposited anywhere in the respiratory system including the nose and mouth. Respirable particles are smaller (10-micron diameter or smaller) and can penetrate deeper into the respiratory system. However, more research is needed to determine the specific properties and particle sizes of carbon black that relate to toxicity. In addition, pulmonary inflammation is an acute effect; more research is needed to determine whether repeated exposures to carbon black could lead to chronic health effects. This new research could lead to revised occupational exposure limits. More information on OELs is provided in the Appendix.

Conclusions

One employee had an elevated BLL and clinical signs consistent with lead toxicity which were likely caused by exposure to lead at work. BLLs in other employees had not been evaluated. We did not see evidence of ongoing water damage or water infiltration. However, past reports of water intrusion and mold growth could have contributed to upper respiratory and eye irritation symptoms reported by some employees. The HVAC system on the second floor was out of balance. The ventilation system for the firing range had deficiencies that could result in employee exposure to gun emissions (including lead) in the range and garage area. We found lead contamination in the garage and illicit drug contamination in the property room. Chemical exposures from criminology techniques were below applicable OELs, but are likely to vary depending on the type and amount of evidence being processed. Implementing the recommendations below will help reduce exposures and improve working conditions at the police department.

Recommendations

On the basis of our findings, we recommend the actions listed below. We encourage the police department to use a labor-management health and safety committee or working group to discuss our recommendations and develop an action plan. Those involved in the work can best set priorities and assess the feasibility of our recommendations for the specific situation at the police department.

Our recommendations are based on an approach known as the hierarchy of controls (see Appendix for more information). This approach groups actions by their likely effectiveness in reducing or removing hazards. In most cases, the preferred approach is to eliminate hazardous materials or processes and install engineering controls to reduce exposure or shield employees. Until such controls are in place, or if they are not effective or feasible, administrative measures and personal protective equipment may be needed.

Elimination and Substitution

Eliminating or substituting hazardous processes or materials reduces hazards and protects employees more effectively than other approaches. Prevention through design, considering elimination or substitution when designing or developing a project, reduces the need for additional controls in the future.

1. Use jacketed or non-lead bullets and lead-free primer when firing guns in a firing range [NIOSH 2009].

Engineering Controls

Engineering controls reduce employees' exposures by removing the hazard from the process or by placing a barrier between the hazard and the employee. Engineering controls protect employees effectively without placing primary responsibility of implementation on the employee.

1. Redesign the firing range or use another firing range that meets all the recommended design elements in the NIOSH Alert titled "Preventing Occupational Exposures to Lead and Noise at Indoor Firing Ranges" [NIOSH 2009]. Do not use the firing range at the department unless it has been redesigned. Proper ventilation is necessary even when lead-free ammunition is used because other potentially harmful metal particulate can be produced when firing such ammunition depending on the makeup of the bullet.

2. Determine change-out schedules for the filters used in the cyanoacrylate fuming chamber, exhaust hood, fingerprint powder downdraft table, and HEPA vacuum. The manufacturers of these systems may have recommended change-out schedules. The carbon bed filters, in particular, should be changed before they become saturated to prevent the release of organic compounds (including ethyl cyanoacrylate) into the atmosphere.

3. Have the exhaust hood in the crime lab tested and certified annually.

4. Hire a contractor to balance the HVAC system on the second floor and provide conditioned air to maintain a relative humidity at or below 60% in the offices and the property room throughout the year. This will help keep occupants comfortable and help reduce the potential for mold growth in these areas.

Administrative Controls

The term "administrative controls" refers to employer-dictated work practices and policies to reduce or prevent hazardous exposures. Their effectiveness depends on employer commitment and employee acceptance. Regular monitoring and reinforcement are necessary to ensure that policies and procedures are followed consistently. Administrative controls are organized below by the work area where the controls primarily apply.

Firing Range

1. Conduct full-shift personal air sampling for lead and other metals (depending on the makeup of the bullets) in the redesigned firing range or another firing range being used and adjacent work areas on days during which multiple firearm shootings are performed consistently throughout the shift. The sampling results for lead will determine which specific elements of the OSHA lead standard [29 CFR 1910.1025] to follow, such as the need for BLL surveillance. The sampling results for other metals should be compared to applicable OELs.

2. Follow the guidance described in the OSHA lead standard [29 CFR 1910.1025]. This standard provides requirements for exposure monitoring, work practices, engineering controls, personal protective equipment, housekeeping, and medical surveillance among other requirements to reduce occupational exposures to lead.

3. Require the bomb team to wear full-body protective clothing (such as the Tyvek® suits worn in the past), nitrile gloves, and a minimum of a NIOSH-approved N95 half-mask filtering facepiece respirator when cleaning the bullet trap with the HEPA vacuum. This team (while wearing the recommended personal protective equipment) should also replace the HEPA filter in the vacuum according to a schedule. Have this team bag and seal the HEPA filter (when it is ready to be changed) and other lead-contaminated materials (including their personal protective equipment) and dispose of these items according to environmental regulations. Following these procedures should protect the bomb team from being exposed to lead. The bomb team employees should be included in a written respiratory protection program that adheres to the OSHA respiratory protection standard [29 CFR 1910.134].

4. Measure noise exposures on officers when they use the redesigned firing range or another firing range. Audiograms should be done annually if their full-shift time-weighted average exposure level is $\geq$ 85 A-weighted decibels [29 CFR 1910.95]. In addition, we recommend following the U.S. Army guideline of performing annual audiometric testing when employees are exposed to air concentrations of lead (or other ototoxicants) $\geq$ 50% of the most protective OEL [U.S. Army 2009]. The NIOSH, OSHA, and ACGIH exposure limit for lead is 50 $\mu g/m^3$ [NIOSH 2010; ACGIH 2013]. If an audiogram indicates a standard threshold shift (compared to baseline levels), the officer should be referred for a medical evaluation.

Parking Garage

1. Sample surfaces (1 square foot in area) that employees regularly contact (in the garage and other areas of the police department) using NIOSH Method 9100 [NIOSH 2010] to ensure that the surfaces are "free as practicable of accumulations of lead" according to the OSHA lead standard [29 CFR 1910.1025(h)(l)]. The discussion section provides more information on OSHA's interpretation of "free as practicable of accumulations of lead." Our surface sampling locations and results (Table 3) can be used to guide your sampling plan. Surfaces that are not "free as practicable of accumulations of lead" should be cleaned and resampled. A variety of cleaners have been shown to be effective at removing lead dust on surfaces [EPA 1997; Lewis et al. 2006; Lewis et al. 2012]. A more aggressive cleaner may be needed for the mixture of lead and grime on the floor of the garage. Employees who do the cleaning should wear protective full-body clothing and gloves that are resistant to the cleaners. The clothing, gloves, and consumable cleaning items should be disposed of according to environmental regulations.

2. Instruct employees to remove work shoes before entering their home and to store them in an area inaccessible to children. Officers who walk through the parking garage at the police department could contaminate the bottom of their shoes with lead. Keeping work shoes out of the home and out of reach of children should reduce the potential for exposing family members to lead.

Property Room

1. Clean the surfaces inside the property room routinely. A vacuum equipped with a HEPA filter can be used to clean porous and nonporous surfaces. Environmentally friendly cleaners and disposable paper towels can be used for all other nonporous surfaces. Because there are no regulations regarding what can be labeled "environmentally friendly," management will need to become knowledgeable about what cleaning materials are appropriate. Useful sources of information to help select the safest products include the National Institutes of Health database at http://householdproducts.nlm.nih.gov/ and the Greenguard Environmental Institute at http://www.greenguard.org/. Employees performing the cleaning should wear protective equipment (gloves, safety glasses) as recommended by the manufacturers of the chosen cleaners.

2. Dry marijuana and other plant-based drugs prior to storage to reduce odors and the potential for mold growth. If possible, seal drug evidence in plastic bags to minimize drug particle or odor releases.

Crime Lab

1. Develop a written crime lab health and safety plan that describes workplace hazards, standard operating procedures, engineering controls, and personal protective equipment required for each method officers use to process evidence. For guidance, refer to the International Association for Identification, *Safety Guidelines* [IAI 2004] and the Federal Bureau of Investigation, *Handbook of Forensic Services* [FBI 2007]. This plan should be updated regularly (e.g., annually) or as needed.

2. Conduct full-shift personal air sampling for carbon black during fingerprint dusting at a crime scene that requires several hours of processing. These sampling results will provide greater confidence that exposure under actual field conditions are below the applicable OELs.

Second Floor Offices

1. Inspect the second floor plenum and department roof periodically for active water intrusion. Repair any leaks and dry any water damaged porous materials within 24–48 hours to prevent mold growth. If they cannot be dried within this time period they should be replaced.

All Areas of the Police Department

1. Wash hands thoroughly after performing work in the firing range, garage, property room, crime lab, or crime scene. This is especially important to do before eating, drinking, or smoking to prevent potential hand to mouth transmission and ingestion of chemical contaminants. Hands should be washed with soap and water or cleaned with lead decontamination wipes after shooting, handling spent cartridge cases, cleaning weapons, or doing other work that could result in hand contact with lead-contaminated surfaces (even if gloves are worn).

Personal Protective Equipment

Personal protective equipment is the least effective means for controlling hazardous exposures. Proper use of personal protective equipment requires a comprehensive program and a high level of employee involvement and commitment. The right personal protective equipment must be chosen for each hazard. Supporting programs such as training, change-out schedules, and medical assessment may be needed. Personal protective equipment should not be the sole method for controlling hazardous exposures. Rather, personal protective equipment should be used until effective engineering and administrative controls are in place.

1. Wear nitrile gloves when cleaning firearms, handling spent cartridge cases, handling illicit drug evidence, performing criminology procedures, or when doing work in the garage or firing range that could result in lead contamination on the hands. If the automotive maintenance employee works under vehicles (on the floor of the garage), this employee should be given disposable coveralls or coveralls that are kept at work and laundered periodically (e.g., weekly) by a professional service.

2. Use double hearing protection (earmuffs and ear plugs) for impulsive noise generated during weapons firing [NIOSH 2009].

3. Provide employees who voluntarily use N95 filtering facepiece respirators during fingerprint dusting with a copy of Appendix D, "Information for Employees Using Respirators When Not Required Under the Standard," of the OSHA respiratory protection standard [29 CFR 1910.134].

Appendix: Occupational Exposure Limits and Health Effects

NIOSH investigators refer to mandatory (legally enforceable) and recommended OELs for chemical, physical, and biological agents when evaluating workplace hazards. OELs have been developed by federal agencies and safety and health organizations to prevent adverse health effects from workplace exposures. Generally, OELs suggest levels of exposure that most employees may be exposed to for up to 10 hours per day, 40 hours per week, for a working lifetime, without experiencing adverse health effects. However, not all employees will be protected if their exposures are maintained below these levels. Some may have adverse health effects because of individual susceptibility, a pre-existing medical condition, or hypersensitivity (allergy). In addition, some hazardous substances act in combination with other exposures, with the general environment, or with medications or personal habits of the employee to produce adverse health effects. Most OELs address airborne exposures, but some substances can be absorbed directly through the skin and mucous membranes.

Most OELs are expressed as a time-weighted average exposure. A time-weighted average refers to the average exposure during a normal 8- to 10-hour workday. Some chemical substances and physical agents have recommended short-term exposure limit or ceiling values. Unless otherwise noted, the short-term exposure limit is a 15-minute time-weighted average exposure. It should not be exceeded at any time during a workday. The ceiling limit should not be exceeded at any time.

In the United States, OELs have been established by federal agencies, professional organizations, state and local governments, and other entities. Some OELs are legally enforceable limits; others are recommendations.

- The U.S. Department of Labor OSHA permissible exposure limits (29 CFR 1910 [general industry]; 29 CFR 1926 [construction industry]; and 29 CFR 1917 [maritime industry]) are legal limits. These limits are enforceable in workplaces covered under the Occupational Safety and Health Act of 1970.

- NIOSH recommended exposure limits are recommendations based on a critical review of the scientific and technical information and the adequacy of methods to identify and control the hazard. NIOSH recommended exposure limits are published in the *NIOSH Pocket Guide to Chemical Hazards* [NIOSH 2010]. NIOSH also recommends risk management practices (e.g., engineering controls, safe work practices, employee education/training, personal protective equipment, and exposure and medical monitoring) to minimize the risk of exposure and adverse health effects.

- Other OELs commonly used and cited in the United States include the threshold limit values, which are recommended by the American Conference of Governmental Industrial Hygienists, a professional organization, and the workplace environmental exposure levels, which are recommended by the American Industrial Hygiene

Association, another professional organization. The threshold limit values and workplace environmental exposure levels are developed by committee members of these associations from a review of the published, peer-reviewed literature. These OELs are not consensus standards. Threshold limit values are considered voluntary exposure guidelines for use by industrial hygienists and others trained in this discipline "to assist in the control of health hazards" [ACGIH 2013]. Workplace environmental exposure levels have been established for some chemicals "when no other legal or authoritative limits exist" [AIHA 2011].

Outside the United States, OELs have been established by various agencies and organizations and include legal and recommended limits. The Institut für Arbeitsschutz der Deutschen Gesetzlichen Unfallversicherung (Institute for Occupational Safety and Health of the German Social Accident Insurance) maintains a database of international OELs from European Union member states, Canada (Québec), Japan, Switzerland, and the United States. The database, available at http://www.dguv.de/ifa/en/gestis/limit_values/index.jsp, contains international limits for more than 1,500 hazardous substances and is updated periodically.

OSHA requires an employer to furnish employees a place of employment free from recognized hazards that cause or are likely to cause death or serious physical harm [Occupational Safety and Health Act of 1970 (Public Law 91–596, sec. 5(a)(1))]. This is true in the absence of a specific OEL. It also is important to keep in mind that OELs may not reflect current health-based information.

When multiple OELs exist for a substance or agent, NIOSH investigators generally encourage employers to use the lowest OEL when making risk assessment and risk management decisions. NIOSH investigators also encourage use of the hierarchy of controls approach to eliminate or minimize workplace hazards. This includes, in order of preference, the use of (1) substitution or elimination of the hazardous agent, (2) engineering controls (e.g., local exhaust ventilation, process enclosure, dilution ventilation), (3) administrative controls (e.g., limiting time of exposure, employee training, work practice changes, medical surveillance), and (4) personal protective equipment (e.g., respiratory protection, gloves, eye protection, hearing protection). Control banding, a qualitative risk assessment and risk management tool, is a complementary approach to protecting employee health. Control banding focuses on how broad categories of risk should be managed. Information on control banding is available at http://www.cdc.gov/niosh/topics/ctrlbanding/. This approach can be applied in situations where OELs have not been established or can be used to supplement existing OELs.

References

ACGIH [2001]. Ethyl cyanoacrylate. In: Documentation of the threshold limit values and biological exposure indices. Cincinnati, OH: American Conference of Governmental Industrial Hygienists.

ACGIH [2011]. Carbon black. In: Documentation of the threshold limit values and biological exposure indices. Cincinnati, OH: American Conference of Governmental Industrial Hygienists.

ACGIH [2013]. Threshold limit values for chemical substances and physical agents and biological exposure indices. Cincinnati, OH: American Conference of Governmental Industrial Hygienists.

AIHA [2010]. Facts about mold. Falls Church, VA: American Industrial Hygiene Association. [http://www.aiha.org/get-involved/VolunteerGroups/Documents/BiosafetyVG-FactsAbout%20MoldDecember2011.pdf]. Date accessed: July 2013.

AIHA [2011]. Emergency response planning guidelines and worplace environmental exposure levels. Fairfax, VA: American Industrial Hygiene Association (AIHA).

ASHRAE [2007]. Justice facilities. In: 2007 ASHRAE handbook: heating, ventilating, and air-conditioning applications. Atlanta, GA: American Society of Heating, Refrigerating and Air-Conditioning Engineers, Inc.

Brown-Williams H, Lichterman J, Kosnett M [2009]. Indecent exposure: lead puts workers and families at risk. Health Research in Action, University of California, Berkeley. Perspectives 4(1):1–9.

California Department of Public Health, Occupational Lead Poisoning Prevention Program [2009]. Medical guidelines for the lead-exposed worker. [http://www.cdph.ca.gov/programs/olppp/Documents/medgdln.pdf]. Date accessed: July 2013.

CDC (Centers for Disease Control and Prevention) [2012]. Update on blood lead levels in children. [http://www.cdc.gov/nceh/lead/ACCLPP/blood_lead_levels.htm]. Date accessed: July 2013.

CDC (Centers for Disease Control and Prevention) [2013]. Fourth national report on human exposure to environmental chemicals, Updated Tables, March, 2013. [http://www.cdc.gov/exposurereport/pdf/FourthReport_UpdatedTables_Mar2013.pdf]. Date accessed: July 2013.

CFR. Code of Federal Regulations. Washington, DC: U.S. Government Printing Office, Office of the Federal Register.

Chan PC, Ho KH, Kan KK, Stuhmiller JH, Mayorga MA [2001]. Evaluation of impulse noise criteria using human volunteer data. J Acoust Soc Am 110(4):1967–1975.

CSTE [2009]. Public health reporting and national notification for elevated blood lead levels. CSTE position statement 09-OH-02. Atlanta, GA: Council of State and Territorial Epidemiologists. [http://c.ymcdn.com/sites/www.cste.org/resource/resmgr/PS/09-OH-02.pdf]. Date accessed: July 2013.

EPA [1997]. Laboratory study of lead-cleaning efficacy. Washington, DC: U.S. Environmental Protection Agency, Office of Pollution Prevention and Toxics. EPA 747-R-97-002.

EPA [2009]. Residential air cleaners (second edition): a summary of available information. [http://www.epa.gov/iaq/pubs/residair.html#Air_Filters_-_Available_Guidance_for_Their_Comparison]. Date accessed: July 2013.

FBI [2007]. Crime scene safety. In: Waggoner K, ed. Handbook of foresnic services. Quantico, VA: U.S. Federal Bureau of Investigation, Laboratory Division, pp. 147–169.

HUD [2012]. Guidelines for evaluation and control of lead-based paint hazards in housing, 2nd ed. In: U.S. Department of Housing and Urban Development, Office of Healthy Homes and Lead Hazard Control. [http://portal.hud.gov/hudportal/HUD?src=/program_offices/healthy_homes/lbp/hudguidelines]. Date accessed: July 2013.

Hwang YH, Chiang HY, Yen-Jean MC, Wang JD [2009]. The association between low levels of lead in blood and occupational noise-induced hearing loss in steel workers. Sci Total Environ *408*(1):43–49.

IAI (International Association for Identification) [2004]. Safety guidelines: second edition. [http://www.theiai.org/publications/]. Date accessed: July 2013.

Kosnett M, Wedeen R, Rothberg S, Hipkins K, Materna B, Schwartz B, Hu H, Woolf A [2007]. Recommendations for medical management of adult lead exposure. Environ Health Perspect *115*(3):463–471.

Kardous CA, Willson RD, Hayden CS, Szlapa P, Murphy WJ, Reeves ER [2003]. Noise exposure assessment and abatement strategies at an indoor firing range. Appl Occup Environ Hyg *18*(8):629–636.

Lai H, Corbin I, Almirall JR [2008]. Headspace sampling and detection of cocaine, MDMA, and marijuana via volatile markers in the presence of potential interferences by solid phase microextraction-ion mobility spectrometry (SPME-IMS). Anal Bioanal Chem *392*(1–2):105–113.

Lewis RD, Condoor S, Batek J, Ong KH, Backer D, Sterling D, Siria J, Chen JJ, Ashley P [2006]. Removal of lead contaminated dusts from hard surfaces. Environ Sci Technol *40*(2):590–594.

Lewis RD, Ong KH, Emo B, Kennedy J, Brown CA, Condoor S, Thummalakunta L [2012]. Do new wipe materials outperform traditional lead dust cleaning methods? J Occup Environ Hyg 9(8):524–533.

Moline JM, Landrigan PJ [2005]. Lead. In: Rosenstock L, Cullen MR, Brodkin CA, Redlich CA, eds. Textbook of clinical occupational and environmental medicine. 2nd ed. Philadelphia, PA: Elsevier Saunders, pp. 967–979.

Murphy WJ, Tubbs RL [2007]. Assessment of noise exposure for an indoor and outdoor firing range. J Occup Env Hyg 4(9):688–697.

NAMSDL [2008]. State feasibility-based standards. Alexandria, VA: National Alliance for Model State Drug Laws (NAMSDL). [http://www.namsdl.org/library/80C05418-1C23-D4F9-74AF7EFE43761A50/]. Date accessed: July 2013.

NIOSH [2001]. Work-related hearing loss. Cincinnati, OH: U.S. Department of Health and Human Services, Centers for Disease Control and Prevention, National Institute for Occupational Safety and Health, DHHS (NIOSH) Publication No. 2001-103.

NIOSH [2003]. Health hazard evaluation report: Fort Collins Police Services – Fort Collins, Colorado. By Tubbs R and Murphy WJ. Cincinnati, OH: U.S. Department of Health and Human Services, Centers for Disease Control and Prevention, National Institute for Occupational Safety and Health, NIOSH HETA Report No. 2002-0131-2898.

NIOSH [2009]. NIOSH alert: preventing occupational exposure to lead and noise at indoor firing ranges. Cincinnati, OH: U.S. Department of Health and Human Services, Centers for Disease Control and Prevention, National Institute for Occupational Safety and Health, DHHS (NIOSH) Publication No. 2009-136.

NIOSH [2010]. NIOSH pocket guide to chemical hazards. Barsen ME, ed. Cincinnati, OH: U.S. Department of Health and Human Services, Centers for Disease Control and Prevention, National Institute for Occupational Safety and Health, DHHS (NIOSH) Publication No. 2010-168c. [http://www.cdc.gov/niosh/npg/]. Date accessed: July 2013.

NIOSH [2011]. Health hazard evaluation report: evaluation of police officers' exposures to chemicals while working inside a drug vault – Kentucky. By Fent KW, Durgam S, West C, Gibbins J, Smith J. Cincinnati, OH: U.S. Department of Health and Human Services, Centers for Disease Control and Prevention, National Institute for Occupational Safety and Health, NIOSH HETA Report No. 2010-0017-3133.

NIOSH [2013]. NIOSH manual of analytical methods. 4th ed. Schlecht PC, O'Connor PF, eds. Cincinnati, OH: U.S. Department of Health and Human Services, Centers for Disease Control and Prevention, National Institute for Occupational Safety and Health, DHHS (NIOSH) Publication No. 94-113 (August 1994); 1st Supplement Publication 96-135, 2nd Supplement Publication 98-119, 3rd Supplement Publication 2003-154. [http://www.cdc.gov/niosh/docs/2003-154/].

OSHA [1985]. OSHA Method 55: methyl-2-cyanoacrylate and ethyl-2-cyanoacrylate. In: Sampling and analytical methods. Salt Lake City, Utah: U.S. Department of Labor, Occupational Safety and Health Administration, Organic Methods Evaluation Branch. [http://www.osha.gov/dts/sltc/methods/index.html].

OSHA [2003]. Standard interpretation letter: lead standard 29 CFR 1926.62(i)(2)(ii). [http://www.osha.gov/pls/oshaweb/owadisp.show_document?p_table=INTERPRETATIONS&p_id=25617]. Date accessed: July 2013.

Schwartz BS, Hu H [2007]. Adult lead exposure: time for change. Environ Health Perspect *115*(3):451–454.

Schwartz BS, Stewart WF [2007]. Lead and cognitive function in adults: a question and answers approach to a review of the evidence for cause, treatment, and prevention. Int Rev Psychiatry *19*(6):671–692.

Smith J, Sammons D, Robertson S, Biagini R, Snawder J [2010]. Measurement of multiple drugs in urine, water, and on surfaces using fluorescence covalent microbead immunosorbent assay. Toxicol Mech Methods *20*(9):587–593.

U.S. Army [2009]. Just the facts: occupational ototoxins (ear poisons) and hearing loss. Hearing Conservation and Industrial Hygiene and Medical Safety Management. [http://www.nmcphc.med.navy.mil/downloads/occmed/toolbox/occupationalototoxinfactsheet-chppm.pdf]. Date accessed: July 2013.

Ward EM, Schulte PA, Straif K, Hopf NB, Caldwell JC, Carreon T, DeMarini DM, Fowler BA, Goldstein BD, Hemminki K, Hines CJ, Pursiainen KH, Kuempel E, Lewtas J, Lunn RM, Lynge E, McElvenny DM, Muhle H, Nakajima T, Robertson LW, Rothman N, Ruder AM, Schubauer-Berigan MK, Siemiatycki J, Silverman D, Smith MT, Sorahan T, Steenland K, Stevens RG, Vineis P, Zahm SH, Zeise L, Cogliano VJ [2010]. Research recommendations for selected IARC-classified agents. Environ Health Perspect *118*(10):1355–1362.

Keywords: North American Industry Classification System 922120 (Police Protection), lead, firing range, ventilation, noise, property room, evidence, illicit drugs, mold, indoor environmental quality, criminology procedures, fingerprint dusting, cyanoacrylate fuming

The Health Hazard Evaluation Program investigates possible health hazards in the workplace under the authority of Section 20(a)(6) of the Occupational Safety and Health Act of 1970, 29 U.S.C. 669(a)(6). The Health Hazard Evaluation Program also provides, upon request, technical assistance to federal, state, and local agencies to control occupational health hazards and to prevent occupational illness and disease. Regulations guiding the Program can be found in Title 42, Code of Federal Regulations, Part 85; Requests for Health Hazard Evaluations (42 CFR 85).

Acknowledgments

Analytical Support: Bureau Veritas North America
Desktop Publisher: Mary Winfree
Editor: Ellen Galloway
Health Communicator: Stefanie Brown
Industrial Hygiene Field Assistance: Catherine Beaucham and Jung Ho Choi
Logistics: Donnie Booher and Karl Feldmann

Availability of Report

This report is available at http://www.cdc.gov/niosh/hhe/reports/pdfs/2012-0083-3189.pdf.

Recommended citation for this report:
NIOSH [2013]. Health hazard evaluation report: evaluation of employee exposure to lead and other chemicals at a police department. By Fent KW, Gibbins J, Niemeier T. Cincinnati, OH: U.S. Department of Health and Human Services, Centers for Disease Control and Prevention, National Institute for Occupational Safety and Health, NIOSH HETA Report No. 2012-0083-3189.